Marketing Chiropractic to Medical Doctors

Your Step-by-Step Guide to Increasing Referrals

Jeff Langmaid, DC

Dedicated to Audrey Elizabeth Langmaid

Contents

INTRODUCTION

From our forefathers who risked prosecution, to the trailblazers in research, chiropractors throughout time have shown a thorough dedication to the art, science, and philosophy of our chosen profession. Most students arrive at chiropractic school with an unsurpassed enthusiasm for the practices and principles of chiropractic. This is often due to a personal experience in which chiropractic care altered the course of either their life, or the life of a close family member.

Unbridled enthusiasm and dedication have helped our profession thrive despite a variety of external and internal obstacles. One obstacle we have yet to overcome, however, is a lack of interdisciplinary referrals. It has been estimated that only 30% of primary care physicians have ever made a formal referral to a chiropractor. Although research shows up to 90% of primary care physicians have been asked about chiropractic by their patients'. Previously, we could look to the American Medical Association's prejudice or perhaps a limited amount peer-reviewed research to justify this unfortunate statistic. Now, we must look inward and seek to develop the skills necessary to promote our profession while developing referral relationships with the other physicians in our communities.

For low back pain alone, over half of the visits for treatment are to a primary care physician. This is despite the fact that "treatments commonly recommended by primary care physicians are often highly guideline discordant,...". With a wealth of high-quality peer-reviewed research supporting the efficacy and safety of our care, and many medical doctors unaware of the past dogma of their profession; it becomes clear that scant interdisciplinary referrals are the result of underdeveloped relationships.

Relationships are at the heart of referrals. Professional relationships are built on trust, rapport, clinical expertise, and patient outcomes. Through The Evidence Based Chiropractor, I have been at the forefront of developing and implementing effective, affordable, and elegant interdisciplinary relationship building tools for chiropractors.

I practice with one of the largest spine groups in the world and this has given me unique insight into the referral habits and patterns of medical doctors. In short, I have found what works and what doesn't work.

In this book, you will learn the key components to building these relationships. You will start by establishing some protocols and procedures in your own office. Next, a carefully constructed target list will be created and verified. Then, your MD Meetings will be scheduled, prepared for, and executed. While your success does not hinge solely on the meeting, it can act as a significant referral accelerator. After that, some low maintenance monthly follow up should put you in a position to be the trusted chiropractor for many local physicians.

By systematically reaching out in an elegant, professional, and educational manner; you will be able to position yourself as the local leader and expert in musculoskeletal care. Establishing yourself as the trusted expert while expanding your professional network will create a potent combination for increasing your referrals. The foundation of this technique is learning how you can serve others. As chiropractors, we are excited about the wonders of our care. However, to gain referrals from other providers it is imperative to serve THEIR needs. Fortunately, one of their biggest needs is the ability to help their patients who may be suffering from spine related complaints. The research unequivocally illustrates that primary care providers are woefully undertrained and generally ineffective at treating patients with spine related complaints/pathology. So by learning about their practice, you will be able to position yours.

The core of your outreach should be with monthly research updates. I highly recommend using the fully customized monthly Research Briefs offered by The Evidence Based Chiropractor. These are elegantly customized and white-labeled for your practice. Let us save you the time and energy of scouring research articles by producing the briefs for you. In short, the research briefs should highlight a high-quality piece of relevant research for the targeted physician. We have found that a single page format with a combination of graphics, quotes, and an actionable paragraph framing the importance of the highlighted article will create the most impact. There are a few other ways to bolster your creditability and build trust that can really put the efficacy of the briefs into overdrive. A great way to enhance and accelerate your relationship (and ultimately, referrals) is to set up your MD Meetings.

Setting up and properly executing an MD Meeting is very straightforward if you are prepared. As you will learn, there are a few key points which you will want to address with each health care provider. Included is a conversation about the biggest hurdles to referrals and setting expectations about your care and communication. You will see that a "Socratic" method is best during the remainder of the conversation. This enables you to specifically establish where and when you can provide value and expertise for the care of their patients. For instance, many medical doctors either refer to physical therapy, prescribe medications, or refer to an orthopedist for all spine complaints. As a matter of fact, these 3 simple choices typically make up 99% of their algorithm/treatment protocols. In this book you will see how a referral to your office has distinct advantages over those other options.

For some of us this may seem like a daunting task. However, with this book I have laid out the steps in a systematic and efficient manner which even the most introverted of chiropractors will be able to use for their success. Using a step by step process, you will be able to position yourself in the best manner possible and present yourself "on your terms".

"I AM PLEASED TO ANNOUNCE THAT WE HAVE
DOUBLED OUR DIRECT MD REFERRALS SINCE
IMPLEMENTING YOUR PLAN."
- GOLDI JACQUES-MAYNES, DC

CHAPTER ONE
Why Should I Build Referral Relationships?

Primary care physicians have extremely limited treatment options for musculoskeletal complaints. They truly do not have the tools or expertise necessary to take care of these patients in the best manner possible. Research has shown time and time again that primary care physicians tend to over-prescribe, improperly refer, and over-utilize diagnostics when evaluating spine complaints. As we will learn later, they often use medications as a first line defense. Regardless of our personal thoughts regarding the over-medicalization of our country; there are still a vast amount of people who have contraindications to common anti-inflammatory and pain meds. So what becomes of these patients? Perhaps a referral to physical therapy or a orthopedist? Each of these options have distinct disadvantages for the referring doctor and may even fall against evidence-based guidelines depending upon the suspected condition. Are they currently referred to your office? Research shows chiropractic care to be an appropriate referral for a vast majority of these patients. However, very few physicians blindly refer out of their office. This is where the establishing a relationship built on research is paramount.

Many patients are referred out of their primary care physicians offices without any clear path to better health; only a half hearted script for physical therapy and a prescription for pain medication. Certainly every office is different, but we have all heard a million versions of the same story. "My doc didn't listen to me." "He only came in the room for 15 seconds." "He didn't even examine me." "I knew he was just going to push medications." "I want a solution, not a handful of pills." At this pint we have likely heard this story so many times that we are desensitized to it. There is a better way. Our friends and neighbors are depending on us.

It starts by building referral relationships with these physicians. These relationships have the potential to provide value to their office, your office, and most importantly; a better outcome for the patients. The foundation of your relationship should be research. The WIIFT (whats in it for them) is the bolstering of their own practice reputation (and patient satisfaction) by properly referring patients who receive improvement as a result of that referral.

Referral relationships with other local physicians will help build your reputation and credibility in the community. Additionally, it will create the ability for you to position your practice as a place which is trust worthy and mainstream. With less than 10% of the population seeing a chiropractor, most people do not have personal experience with chiropractic. They instead are forced to rely on the internet, their friends, and their physicians for answers to their questions about chiropractic care. I would venture to say that many physicians would not speak highly of chiropractic care when asked. Otherwise, they would already be referring patients to your office! I would also venture to say that building a professional relationship with your local physicians will greatly influence the way they speak of chiropractic in the future. We may each only be able to play a small part in how chiropractic is viewed on a national or international level, but we can play a huge part in how chiropractic is viewed in our own community. Going to a targeted source of patient referrals (a primary care physician) can have a far greater impact on your practice than a scattershot public marketing campaign.

Another important reason to reach out to physicians in your community is financial. We see many services dedicated to internet and external marketing to the public. Some of these services are fantastic while others leave something to be desired. Either way, external marketing to the public is an essential component of building a chiropractic practice. The challenge of marketing to the public is that it can be difficult to create a target demographic. Essentially, you are targeting ages/incomes/locations without any idea if they have a reason to visit your office. This makes marketing to the public quite inefficient. External marketing to the public is also expensive! Radio spots, billboards, social media, mobile app development, online scheduling; it's enough to make your head spin. Even with careful targeting, this is still a "shotgun" approach. What if you could reach out to a fellow health care professional who had an endless stream of patients who could benefit from our care? You can! It's the medical doctors in your community. We have found that reaching out to medical doctors can be easily added on to your current marketing plan with little added expense. In fact, you should be able to pay for a full year of physician marketing with just a few referred patients.

Finally, and perhaps most importantly, facilitating communication between yourself and other local physicians will inevitably lead to better patient outcomes. By providing educational and informative research updates, you will be assisting those physicians in making better decisions for their patients care. Also, by sending case notes and discharge notes, each patient will have a more complete medical record. Both of these items are imperative as outcomes assessments become a key contributor to reimbursement. By leading the way and providing effective, safe, and cost- effective conservative care the transition from interventional reimbursement to outcome based reimbursement will be much less painful. With fundamentally sound, congruent documentation and a variety of sources for incoming patients- you will be proactively preparing your practice for any unexpected changes in the healthcare landscape.

CHAPTER TWO
Cleaning Your House

Before you begin your outreach, there are a few items you should address in your own office to make sure you maximize your efforts. A couple simple changes to office paperwork has the potential to pay large dividends in your physician marketing.

The good news is that your office more than likely already has a wealth of information to help your physician targeting. Each and every one of your patients should be listing their primary care physicians on their intake paperwork in your office. If you do not have your new patients list their primary care physician on their intake paperwork then I recommend you start collecting that information immediately! It is not only helpful in your external marketing, but also a key component to complete and accurate patient health records as you begin to communicate with their other health care providers. Learning the popular primary care physicians of your patients is crucially important. First, it will provide you with detailed, hyper-targeted information which you can then use to fine tune your target list. Then, it will be much easier to provider social proof of the efficacy of your care as you will read below. You will already with co-managing these patients!

Assuming that you have been collecting this information, now is a great time to put it to use. Getting a feel for the more popular primary care physicians in town, as well as in your office, will help you develop your physician list. Not only does it provide you with information to build your physician list, but it provides opportunity for continued outreach in the form of patient notes. Patient notes are an essential bridge between you and the primary care provider. Please always follow your local, state, and federal laws regarding patient communication and protected health information.

Research has shown that chiropractors are woefully inadequate at the transmission of patient care notes to other doctors. This may be a combination of fear, inadequate documentation, or just being unsure what to send. Fortunately, many primary care physicians are busy and do not want or need a "complete" evaluation note from you office. They are rarely concerned with chiropractic techniques, radiograph listings, specific examination findings, etc. Quite simply, they are interested in four pieces of information.

Pertinent Information for Case Notes

Who   Patient Name and Date of Service

Why   Chief Complaint

What   Diagnosis

How   Treatment Plan and Goals

Who- What is the patients name and when did they visit your office?

Why- Why is the patient in your office? Just a simple line or two regarding their chief complaint will do.

What- What is the condition? List your diagnosis codes as determined by your history, evaluation, and imaging (if applicable).

How- How is the patient expected to improve? Let them know your anticipated treatment plan and goals.

Most EHR/EMR's can actually export this data automatically! However, if you need to perform this manually, a simple template will make this a painless and easy process.

By providing case notes to your patients primary care physicians, you are most importantly assisting them in keeping an accurate and complete health care record. Additionally, you are able to get your name in front of the primary care physician and establish common ground. They will know that you are actively treating their patients and providing communication in a professional manner. Also, they will be able to track and see how patients improve in your office, providing them with valuable "proof" that chiropractic care can benefit their patients!

You do not need to inundate these physicians with notes, but sending notes after the initial evaluation and at their discharge from active care is a good protocol. It is important to note the phrase ACTIVE care. The patient may choose to continue in your office on a wellness/maintenance schedule. This type of care does not necessarily require updates to the referral physician. In my opinion, ACTIVE care is why the patient was referred, and why the notes are imperative. When a patient advances to wellness/maintenance care it is a decision between them and you and no updates are necessary, until they again enter active care.

Jeff Langmaid

CHAPTER THREE
Building Your Target List

So you have made the decision (a wise one) to begin outreach to medical doctors in your town. Building your physician list is the first step towards creating a consistent and sustained outreach program in your circle of practice. I highly recommend downloading the free Evidence Based Chiropractor Monthly Tracking Sheet at our website. This sheet keeps your contacts tidy and allows you a quick glance at your progress during the year.

Your marketing and outreach will only be as effective as the list you are using. Determining not only the number of doctors on your list, but the types of doctors, is crucial. I highly recommend having 50 physicians on your list. For some of you in rural areas, 50 doctors may be extending 10 miles of more from your practice. While others, in more urban environments may have 50 doctors within three or four blocks. For those of us in the suburbs, a list of 50 doctors within five to seven miles of your practice will be easily attainable. If you can afford to maintain an active marketing list of 100 physicians, then go for it! A larger list will produce greater results (as long as it's still highly targeted). However, my members have found that a list of 50 physicians provides the coverage, diversity, and reach necessary to begin building referral relationships.

There are three great resources to curate your list. The first is the WebMD physician search. They make it easy to search by specialty and location while retaining a high-quality and thorough list. WebMD physician search is a key piece to creating your list. Two other search engines include the ZocDoc search and a good old fashioned Google search. Also, keep your eyes peeled during your daily travels around town. There very well may be a few doctors offices which you have passed hundreds of times but never "noticed" before. (Also, do not forget obtaining the names of popular primary care physicians in your area from your current patients.)

WebMD

ZocDoc

Google

The types of specialists I recommend reaching out to include Primary Care Physicians, Internists, Family Physician, Orthopedic Surgeon, Neurologist, OB/GYN and Pediatricians. You will tailor this list depending upon your practice style.

Primary Care Physicians should make up 50-75% of your list. They are important referral partners for a few reasons. First, up to 30% of their daily practice volume is directly related to spine complaints. Also, they have extremely limited options for treating these conditions. Finally, the options which they do have are generally ineffective and not included in current evidence-based guidelines.

Your Practice	Your Target Specialty
Pediatric	Pediatricians
Sports	Sports Medicine, Extremity Specialists
Geriatric	Internal Medicine/Urgent Care
Pregnancy	OB/GYN, Midwife, Doula
Family Care	Pediatricians, OB/GYN, Primary Care
Relief Care	Primary Care, Internal Medicine, Urgent Care

The remaining portion of your list can be a mix of specialists. Your choice of specialists should correspond to your personal practice style. It may be a focus on pediatrics or perhaps sports medicine. It is best to take an unbiased look at your practice layout, systems, staff, and skill set to match your "niche" interests with your specialist outreach. For instance, spending time and money reaching out to pediatricians would not be a good idea if you office is laid out for sports medicine and rehab.

As you can see, creating your list does not require an abundance of time. Your attention to detail is the key. Focusing and refining your list will drive the efficiency and effectiveness of your outreach. I would use a 5% turnover of the your each quarter as an accurate churn rate. This would be an exchange of 2-3 doctors per quarter. A physician may drop off your list due to lack of interest, practice relocation/consolidation, insurance restrictions limiting direct referral, etc.

CHAPTER FOUR
Verifying Your List

Now that you have a working list, I highly recommend calling the offices to verify the address and doctor. Calling each office individually may seem tedious, and is perhaps one of the more labor intensive tasks in your outreach, but it will pay large dividends to have an accurate and up to date physician list. If you do not, you may end up wasting time, energy, and postage. By verifying your list, you are able to further focus your marketing.

Many primary care physicians are consolidating, forming small group practices, or joining larger groups. Like us, they are facing dwindling reimbursement and increased scrutiny of office documentation. This makes group practice a more desirable situation as they can split overhead and essentially create "power in numbers". For our purposes, it is important to keep in mind this changing practice landscape in relation to our physician list. It is wise to do a broad update of your list once a year, as some offices will have undoubtably added new physicians.

The actually calling of your list can easily be done by your front desk staff. There is no advantage to the doctor making the call because all the information you will need is available from the front desk staff of the office which you are calling.

The goal of this call is simply to verify your information. It should be short and to the point. I recommend the following scripting-

"Good morning, this is John Jones from ABC Spine Clinic. I am calling to confirm your address at 123 Main Street, and also that Dr. Smith is still practicing at your location."

If yes, then a simple "Thank you, have a great day" is sufficient. If the receptionist answers "no" then there are a few options and opportunities. A "no" will either equal a new address (which is important to update) or that Dr. Smith changed offices. This is important because you are then able to ask the new address of Dr. Smith's office, AND you can find out the new physicians name and specialty.

As you go through this process, your list might grow as you discover new physicians practicing in these offices'. It is important to not discard this valuable information, but keep a larger "master list" of physicians in your area. While you may choose to actively market to 50 physicians; if your master list is 100 physicians then it will be easy to replace doctors on your active list as people move, retire, etc.

Consolidating your master list down to your active list is both art and science. Your active list should be 50%-75% primary care and internal medicine doctors. The rest will be physicians who practice in a specialty which aligns with your practice interests. Perhaps you have additional training in pregnancy care and pediatrics. Then you would include a fair amount of OB/GYN's and Pediatricians on your active list. If you are more interested in sports chiropractic then you could include some extremity physicians and sports medicine experts.

Certainly at the top of your active list will be physicians who have previously referred to your practice. These doctors already have a favorable opinion of your practice and your outreach will be focused upon further establishing yourself as their first choice. Next, I believe it's important to create a balance between geographical location in relation to your practice and the volume of patients you have seen which list this doctor as their primary care physician. For instance, you may have a primary care physician who practices in the same office building as you. However, you may notice that many of your patients list a doctor who practices across town as their primary care physician. Ideally, it would be wise to include both physicians on your active list. I tend to lean towards physician's whose name I see more often on my patients intake forms. A doctor in my office complex who sees 10 visits a week and whom I see no patients list as their primary care physician is much less valuable as a marketing target than a doctor across town who sees 100 visits per week and I see 10% of my practice listing as their primary care physician.

When you get towards the end of your list this decision making process can be a bit more challenging. As we touched on earlier; I would expect 2-4% of your list to change each quarter as physicians consolidate, move or retire. There will be constant refinement of the list as your begin to learn about the physicians and their practices. The effectiveness of your list and outreach should continue to build as you refine your list through-out time.

CHAPTER FIVE
Setting Up Meeting's

Meeting your local MD's is a great way to accelerate your relationship for many reasons. Just like your relationships outside of chiropractic; trust, rapport, and communication are most easily managed in person. Establishing a friendly relationship through a brief meeting will enable you to gain a thorough understanding of their practice. With this information you will be able to position yourself in the best way possible to maximize the relationship.

Pharmaceutical companies usually provide the "competition" you have for meeting a doctor at lunch . Thankfully, the government continues to push for greater transparency and hard caps on the pharmaceutical dollars which are given to physicians. Not only is this the right thing to do ethically, but it gives us the ability to have greater access to medical doctors. Some pharmaceutical companies are reducing these expenditures by up to 50%, which will inevitably mean less physician lunches. As they have less opulent pharmaceutical lunches, we are able to schedule meaningful meetings where interdisciplinary communication can be fostered leading to better outcomes for their patients through conservative care. However, some offices will still be booked weeks or months in advance for lunches. Sometimes, you may be fast tracked to meet the doctor because you are not a 'rep' but another physician. Either way, it's important to get started!

Setting up who you are going to meet with should be relatively straight forward. If you are a member of The Evidence Based Chiropractor then you should be working with a list of roughly 50 MD's in your area who are receiving your monthly Research Briefs. This list is a great starting point. If you have already received referrals from an MD in your area then I would move those MD's to the top of the list. Then, I recommend that you sort the remaining offices by size, location, and practice type. Many times smaller offices are easier to get into and have less restriction regarding referrals. Also, offices which are physically closer to your practice will be more appealing than those at the edge of your circle of practice.

I initially aim to set up one meeting per week. Realistically, you are probably not going to call 50 offices and set up 50 meetings. However, you should expect to set up roughly 12-24 meetings. By setting up 1 per week, you are able to set an agenda for a few months at a time, and also have the time to reflect between meetings on what works and what you need to work on.

Later in this chapter you will find my sample script for calling your local MD offices. Feel free to alter the script to fit your practice. It should feel natural and comfortable. This is a great activity to delegate to a member of your staff.

Getting one-on-one time with the doctor generally takes place at one of two encounter types; a traditional lunch meeting or a before/after hours meeting.

Providing lunch for the doctor or staff is not mandatory, however, you will want to make that decision before calling the offices so there is no confusion. If you have the budget to provide lunch, it is a nice gesture and of course, creates a nice appearance. If providing lunch is outside of your budget, the meeting is still extremely valuable. I have found that when I provide lunch, I usually meet most of the staff in addition to the physician. When I have not provided lunch, I have generally just met with the physician. There are advantages and disadvantages to both. It is best to make the decision based on your budget and then move forward from there.

Typically the before/after hours meeting is more casual and there is no expectation of food or beverage.

If you have been in practice more than a few months it is highly likely that you have co-managed (even if you were unaware) some patients with other local physicians. I always like to frame the MD Meeting call in a way which emphasizes the co-management of patients. This makes the flow of the conversations much better and eliminates the feeling of a "cold call". Below you will find a few sample scripts to get started.

If you are booking a lunch-

"Hello, my name is John Jones and I am calling on behalf of Dr. Lang-maid at ABC Spine Clinic. He has co-managed quite a few patients with your doctor but has not had the opportunity to formally introduce himself. He would like to book a lunch at your office. May I speak to your office manager to book a lunch?"

If you are booking a short meeting-

"Hello, my name is John Jones and I am calling on behalf of Dr. Lang-maid at ABC Spine Clinic. He has co-managed quite a few patients with your doctor but has not had the opportunity to formally introduce himself. What is the best day and time for Dr. Langmaid to stop by and meet your doctor? Dr. Langmaid is flexible to stop by directly before or after your clinic hours or he could meet the doctor at lunch."

Generally, they will put you through to the person who books the lunches/ meetings. At this point you can decide on a day/time and ask how many staff members/physicians will be in attendance. Mark all of this information down on your MD Tracking Sheets for future reference. Congrats! You have now booked your first MD Meeting.

Occasionally, the individual you need to speak with with be unavailable. If so, just use the aforementioned script on the answering machine and be sure to leave your office number or cell phone. Make a note of whose answering machine the message was left on along with the date and time.

By finding out how many staff/physicians will be present early in the process (some office may book lunches as much as 3 months out) you will be better prepared for your follow up call a few days before the meeting. Not only will this assist with your preparation of material and research, but you can also make the determination of whether or not you would like to provide a lunch for the staff.

One of the only complications I have run into is that some offices only refer to "preferred providers". This is true, at least in my area, with a large insurance company which has "Gold Plus" plans. I have spent a great deal of time and money at some offices only to find out (after I purchased lunch of course) that they will never refer to me due to their insurance company contracts. The best way to address this is after you contact the lunch booker, but before your settle a date. Ask, "Dr. Jones only other question is whether your office only refers patients to clinicians on a preferred provider list?" If the answer is yes, then it is much better for you to save your money and not provide lunch. A great follow up in that case is, "Fantastic, Dr. Jones prefers to book these appointments himself. Could I have your name and extension so he may contact you?" Then, you can decide whether you want to try to book a one on one meeting or move on to the next office.

Also, provide your staff member making these calls with a "cheat sheet". This should have all the information about your practice that a person on the other end of the line may ask. Some of these items include- address/ location, phone number, fax number, email, website.

CHAPTER SIX
Prep for Success

As you begin to fill up your calendar with meetings it is a good idea to begin your preparation work. Below is a list of the material which I recommend having handy during your meetings.

Your Folder Should Contain the Following

    Introductory Letter

    Practice Information Sheet

    Curriculum Vitae

    Research on Cervical Spine Efficacy

    Research on Lumbar Spine Efficacy

    Research on Cervical Spine Safety

    Chiropractic Cost-Effectiveness Research

    Current Research Brief

A branded folder is an easy, affordable, and elegant way to present your research during the MD Meeting. These can easily be obtained online or through your local print shop. If you order 50-100 of these, you will be well prepared for a variety of meetings without breaking the bank. The front can simply have your practice logo, name, address, phone number, and website. If you are not familiar with graphic design then I recommend you hire a professional to layout the front/back of your folder.

Elegance, professionalism, and creative branding will go a long way and are not to be underestimated. This will be the physicians first "look" at your practice and if it looks like your folders came out of a box from 1905, then they may assume that your treatment matches. Positioning of your practice through high-quality branding is of supreme importance!

The Introductory Letter is what we refer to as the "Ice Breaker Letter" at The Evidence Based Chiropractor. This letter is designed to set up your future follow up (monthly Research Brief), briefly highlight some of the conditions you treat, and address the major 3 major hinderances to referrals. Letting the physician know that you understand the difficulties in keeping up with musculoskeletal research sets the stage for your future monthly outreach through research. This will not only provide educational value for the doctor, but also further position yourself as the leading local authority on musculoskeletal care. Believe it or not, there are some physicians who are still unsure of exactly what a chiropractor does in practice. List a few of the conditions which you are specifically looking for through referrals. This could be as simple as Cervical and Lumbar Pain, Disc Herniations, or even Neuropathy and Pregnancy Related Low Back Pain. Just tailor the list to your practice style.

Finally, it is important to address the 3 major hurdles to referrals. We will address these 3 items in depth in the MD MEETING section of this book. However, in short, they are-

1) A lack of case notes, diagnosis, and treatment plan

2) The belief that patients are pressured into long term care plans

3) The fear that you will "steal" their patients

I simply let the physician know that when they refer a patient they can expect prompt updates on the diagnosis and treatment plan, that all patients receive an initial trial course of care, and that we have found patients receive the best results when their chiropractor and primary care physician are working together.

Other primary items inside of this folder should be your Curriculum Vitae and Practice Information Sheet. The Practice Information Sheet is essentially your practice "one-sheet" as its known in the entertainment industry. This sheet will have your name, logo, phone number, address, website, email, major insurances taken, names of staff, and everything else that the referring physician may need to make the referral process as easy as possible. The referring doctors front desk staff should be able to refer to this single sheet and obtain nearly all the relevant information about your practice at a glance. The importance of a well-done Practice Information Sheet can not be overstated.

Next, you will want to be prepared with some long form research regarding the efficacy of chiropractic care for cervical and lumbar complaints. Often, primary care physicians are unfamiliar with current musculoskeletal research. They may be relying on habit and here-say to make their clinical decisions. A vast majority of the spine complaints which they encounter on a daily basis are of the cervical and lumbar spine. Being prepared with research directly relevant to the efficacy of our care for these complaints is imperative. I favor presenting long form research during the MD Meeting and then following up with the MD Research Briefs each month. The long form research provides great breadth and depth as you establish your relationship. Then, following up each month with your Research Brief will grow and develop the seed of your relationship which was planted during the meeting.

A piece of research citing the safety of adjusting the cervical spine should also be in your folder. Unfortunately, many physicians confuse the profession of Chiropractic with the act of practicing chiropractic. In other words, they believe that everyone who comes through our doors receives a high velocity cervical spine adjustment. When they see a patient in pain with limited ROM, they cannot imagine a high velocity manipulation as a viable treatment and become concerned with its safety. They may have heard a comment or even remember some of the propaganda from before the WILK V. AMA case. At any rate, many physicians are unaware just how safe cervical spine manipulation is, and having the research handy in the face of tough questions is the best way to go. I do not recommend going overboard with your presentation of the safety of cervical spine manipulation. You do not want to appear defensive or give the impression that you are "hiding" something in the research. We all know that the safety of cervical spine manipulation is a delicate topic and subject to controversy. The bottom line is that there are no current studies which show direct causation between cervical spine adjustments and vertebral artery dissection. Handling this topic in a professional and forthright manner will best serve everyones interests.

The final piece of long form research I recommend bringing is on the cost- effectiveness of chiropractic care. There are some physicians who may believe that chiropractic care is expensive and not covered by insurance carriers. It is important to show the cost savings that chiropractic care provides when compared to injections, physical therapy, and surgery.

Your latest Monthly Research Brief should also be included. This gives a nice "preview" as to the content they will receive each month and sets the precedent that you are looking to build a long-term relationships based on the highest quality peer reviewed research.

Business cards and other promotional items can be placed in the bag/folder. The promotional items you create are only limited by your imagination. Many companies provide a plethora of low cost items. Just be sure that your promotional items retain the elegance of your other marketing items while continuing to fall within your brand standards.

Providing referral pads is optional. Some offices will be very interested in using your referral pads (it also keeps present time consciousness when left in their office), while others will either use their own or none at all. Anything you can do to make the referral process as easy and straightforward as possible is beneficial. The doctor should be aware that you have provided referral pads, but you will accept referrals through any means which makes their process easiest.

CHAPTER SEVEN
Counting Down for Launch

Approximately 3 days prior to your scheduled lunch meeting, you should call the office and confirm your engagement. I have two scripts; one for if I am bringing lunch and the other if I am simply meeting the physician. The purpose of this call is to not only confirm your day/time but also to verify the number of attendees and any dietary restrictions (if you are bringing food). Below you will see a few sample scripts for this phone call.

If you are bringing lunch-

"Hello, this is Dr. Langmaid from ABC Spine Clinic. I am scheduled to come into your office during lunch this Thursday at 12:30 pm. I want to confirm the date and time, find out how many people will be attending, and also see if anyone in your office has any dietary restrictions."

If you are not bringing lunch-

"Hello, this is Dr. Langmaid from ABC Spine Clinic. I am scheduled to come to your office at 12:00 this Thursday and meet Dr. Smith. I want to confirm the date and time. Also, if anything comes up Dr. Smith can reach me directly on my cell phone at 123-456-7891."

Most offices are very systematic about their scheduled lunches. This is why in the first example I do not leave my cell phone. Most lunches are scheduled weeks or months out, and they are very particular about making sure everything runs according to plan. However, if you are scheduled to just meet the physician, things can be a little more subject to alteration which is why I typically leave my cell phone number (or office if it's more comfortable for you).

If you decide to provide lunch-

When providing lunch I have found that local, healthy wraps/sandwiches and salads are winners. You should be able to find a local place which will be able to provide a wrap (individual or platter), salad bowl, and individual waters for roughly $5.00 per person. Some of the larger chains tend to creep up to $7-8 per person, so be careful. With local sandwich shops you may also be able to work out a volume discount if you arrange to do quite a few lunches over the course of a few weeks or months. I was able to negotiate a 10% discount with my local shop.

I tend to avoid using restaurants/catering that requires the food to be kept hot or necessitate an elaborate set up. On occasion, I have had lunches start later than expected due to a last minute add-on to the doctor's schedule. In these cases, it's nice to provide wraps because they won't get cold or messy. Using a healthy product is also nice because it subtlety emphasizes the "holistic" component of your practice.

Also, this is a good time to call your local catering/wrap shop and place your order. Most shops require at least 24 hours to prepare the food. Additionally, you want to make sure they have the proper delivery time available. They are generally going to ask for the time, location, and number of people. If the doctor's office provided you with any special delivery/setup instructions then let the caterer know at this time.

If you are not bringing lunch, it may be a good idea to bring a few branded items (pens, pads, etc) or even a box of coffee or bowl of fruit for the office staff. Extending goodwill and leaving something with your name further deepens the impact of your visit. And you never know; while the MD may be slow to refer, the office assistant may be looking for a chiropractor!

CHAPTER EIGHT
Crushing Your MD Meeting

Alright, you have set up the meeting, prepared your material and are now ready to go. Leave plenty of travel time to the office to account for any traffic.

Upon arriving, you should introduce yourself at the front desk and try to meet as many of the staff as possible. You don't need to go overboard, however, making some small talk; offering a smile and handshake can go a long way. Front desk staff tend to be overlooked, so taking a few minutes to introduce yourself can really set a great first impression.

Top priority with your meeting is to establish some rapport, and generally get the physician to have a favorable impression of you (i.e. - they should "like" you). We tend to refer to our "friends" and people whom we have had favorable results with in the past.

More than likely this doctor does not know if patients receive good results in your office, so the starting point is to make a favorable impression. The easiest way to do this is to ask them about their practice. Find out how long they have been in practice, if they reside in the area, etc. This is a great way to build rapport and it also transitions nicely into getting the information you need to maximize the effectiveness of your meeting.

As you continue with your meeting, the questions you ask should give you the information necessary to position yourself as the best referral choice. This is a dynamic process, and you do not want to force an elaborate presentation of the benefits and features of chiropractic on the doctor. By using the Socratic method and asking questions, you can guide the meeting in a way which maximizes the benefit to your practice. This is not extremely complex, but does take patience and the ability to listen and HEAR what the doctor is saying.

First, casually inquire about whether or not they see a lot of spine conditions in their practice. This question will be answered with resounding "yes". As we know, roughly 30% of patients in a primary care physicians office have scheduled an appointment for a spine complaint. Perhaps they also make a statement regarding "how difficult these patients are to treat". When the doctor answers with those statements you are able to get two pieces of extremely important information. First, you now know without a doubt that they have a plethora of patents who would be best served through referral to your office. Second, if they are frustrated with treatment options then you are in a perfect position to add a valued treatment option and provide a service which is beneficial for the patients (and the doctor).

Briefly, inquire about their current treatment protocols for spine conditions. 99% percent of the time they will respond with one of three answers: Medication, physical therapy, or referral to a Orthopedic/Spine Surgeon/ Neurologist. Fortunately, chiropractic care has significant advantages over all three of these current, and most oft used, treatment options. Below we will touch on all three treatment options and discuss a few possible position statements and interactions based on the physicians answers. It is by all means not an exhaustive list, but will provide the framework necessary to feel confident in your conversation.

Many primary care physicians will prescribe medication as a first-line of defense for nearly all spine pain which comes into their office. Discussions regarding our personal views on the over-medicalization are better left for another day. The bottom line is that if you are able to position yourself as a superior alternative, then patients may be able to avoid taking these medications. There are two directions to direct the conversation with the answer of "I generally prescribe NSAID's for that condition".

One way would be to point out that it must be difficult to treat patients who can't take NSAID's, such as those on many of the common prescribed heart medications. Again, you are empathizing with the difficulty of treatment while subtly alluding to a better alternative. You may choose to point out that you have treated many patients with heart conditions who are unable to take NSAID's and have had great results.

Another way to handle this would be to point out that, while many physicians use medication as first line defense, research continues to show that patients under "usual care" by their primary care physician have far superior outcomes when chiropractic care is added. This would be a great time to present that research paper and inquire whether the physician currently co-manages any patients with a chiropractic physician. In this approach you are essentially stating your understanding (while you may not agree) with their treatment option, but also letting them know that research fully supports the addition of your service for superior outcomes.

Physical therapy is also a common first line treatment option for many primary care physicians. We, as chiropractors, have two distinct advantages over physical therapy. First, we have the spinal manipulation or adjustment. Efficacy studies have proven that spinal adjusting is preferred over passive modalities and mobilization. This is easy to address and substantiate with research. However, the more subtle conversation can highlight that you understand referral for physical therapy can place a burden on the physicians front desk as they go through the verification process. And, furthermore, that often patients are not able to see the therapist for at least 2-3 days. Here you can point out the referral to your office requires no verification AND you will be able to see their patients either the same day or within 24 hours (depending on your office policies). This is a HUGE advantage. Most physicians understand that the sooner the patient receives treatment, the sooner they will be out of the pain and the less disability they will have as a result of their condition.

There is one additional bit of information I also like to insert in the conversation. If time is available, I touch on the fact that while chiropractors are the experts in spinal manipulation due to extensive study and training; we also have the capacity to guide the patient on active exercise, etc. I like to emphasize that proper spinal biomechanics should be re-established prior to "strengthening" (i.e. physical therapy). This ensures that the active exercise component is providing the proper support through a full range of motion. Decompressing and establishing proper function of the joint is essential prior to strengthening and active exercise. This is one reason why chiropractic care has performed so well in research when compared to physical therapy for efficacy. While it may seem obvious that decompression and fluid motion should be established prior to a core strengthening protocol, many physicians have not thought this through. Again, this example is supporting the theories that they are comfortable with while also providing additional information that supports your professional care.

Finally, you may encounter a physician who immediate refers all spine complaints to the local surgeon or neurologist. If so, inquire whom these physicians are; you may be able to add them to your target list. To no one's surprise, there are two ways you can address this referral pattern. One, similar to physical therapy, is to point out that you understand the surgeon is quite busy and is booked a few weeks out. Again, the delayed start to treatment may result in a worse outcome. Many physicians are also aware that less than 2% of patients with spine complaints require surgical intervention. You may point out that you have reached out, or intend to reach out, to the surgeon and hope to establish a protocol for conservative care. The primary care physician may feel more comfortable referring to you knowing that, upon evaluation, you will be happy to send the patient to the surgeon if warranted on exam/diagnostics/or after the trial course of care. Becoming a trusted referral partner of both a local orthopedic surgeon and the primary care physicians will lead to practice full of patients who are much more compliant than those who come in due to a coupon in the mail.

Below are three examples outlining your conversation.

Medical Doctor: Many patients with Neck Pain.
Current Treatment Protocol: Treat "In-House" / Prescribe NSAID's

Sample of Potential Current Challenge and Your Chiropractic Advantage: "While NSAID's can be a valuable tool for cervical spine pain; research has shown spinal manipulation to be an effective, safe, and cost-effective treatment option. It must be challenging when you are faced with patients who are unable to take NSAID's due to co-existing conditions or cardiac patients who also are unable to take NSAID's. Often, I have seen patients have fantastic outcomes when co-managed between their medical doctor and myself. Also, you should note that while high velocity adjusting of the cervical spine is extremely safe, we have many chiropractic technique options available that are low velocity. Let me leave this research brief regarding neck pain and manipulation with you to review."

Medical Doctor: Many patients with Low Back Pain
Current Treatment Protocol: Referral to Physical Therapy

Sample of Potential Current Challenge and Your Chiropractic Advantage: "I understand that low back pain has been very difficult for primary care providers to treat. With over 80% of the population suffering from an episode of low back pain and under 2% being surgical, there are a great number of people requiring conservative care of the lumbar spine. A great deal of research has recently been produced showing chiropractic care to be just as, if not more, effective at treating low back pain than physical therapy. Additionally, we don't require your office to have the burden of authorizations, making things easier for you and also making it faster for the patient to begin care. As a matter of fact, I believe active core strength and stability to be an essential component of lumbar spine care. However, research has shown that this is best accomplished after motion has been restored. In my opinion this is why current literature favors chiropractic care over physical therapy for many lumbar spine conditions."

Medical Doctor: Many patients with Lumbar Disk Herniation Current Treatment Protocol: Referral directly to Orthopedist, Neurologist

Sample of Potential Current Challenge and Your Chiropractic Advantage: "For some patients, referral to a orthopedic surgeon is absolutely warranted. Thankfully, less than 2% non-emergency spine complaints require surgical intervention. While I hear about great results from our local orthopedist, his wait time before the first appointment can be several weeks long. With so few of those patients requiring surgical intervention; I would be happy to evaluate any patient whom you feel would benefit from conservative care. Our office strives to retain a few same day appointments for referrals directly from our partner physicians such as yourself. Additionally, I am in the process of reaching out to our local orthopedic surgeon and hope to co- develop some conservative care protocols and algorithms to better facilitate the spine care of our community."

This should be a short and sweet conversation depending upon the amount of time you have with the doctor. You do not want to beat them over the head with chiropractic treatment protocols and techniques. Many of these physicians are not very familiar with chiropractic; so start slowly! However, if they inquire about treatment protocols and technique then by all means dive right in.

The next item I like to address are the "big 3" hinderances to referrals which are also addressed in your MD Introduction Letter. It is essential that you let the physician know the following items-

Big 3 Hinderance to Chiropractic Referral:

Perception of Long Term Treatment Plans

Lack of Interdisciplinary Communication

"Taking" Patients and Treating Outside Our Scope

Hinderance to Chiropractic Referral #1- Long-term treatment plans

Your Position Statement- "Patients do not receive long term treatment plans, but rather a short trial course of care to determine their response to treatment."

This is important because many doctors have heard stories of patients visiting chiropractors for hundreds of visits. You want to be clear that patients in your office receive a trial course of care to determine whether the outcome goals established during the evaluation are being met. If the goals are being met then the patients are encouraged to continue active care until MMI or maximum functional improvement. If the goals are not met then you will discuss additional treatment options and possible referral. Notice that I said ACTIVE care. This means that you may still continue to see patients (if you and the patient agree) on a maintenance basis without compromising the integrity of your promises. Your case notes cover the active care portion of care. At the the conclusion of active care, depending upon the patients personal health goals, they may choose to incorporate periodic maintenance/wellness chiropractic care into their life. If so, this is a decision made between the patient and your office. If or when they return to active care due to injury or symptomatology, you may choose to "start over" with an initial case note to the primary care physician. The length of your trial course of care will of course be determined by the patients condition and any complicating factors. Often, this will be between 6-12 visits. A typical physical therapy referral is for 12 visits; so physicians are comfortable with this amount of visits. This is congruent with chiropractic research which shows the best indication of long term improvement to be short term improvement within the first two weeks of the initiation care.

Hinderance to Chiropractic Referral #2- Lack of Interdisciplinary Communication

Your Position Statement- "Case notes are faxed over upon evaluation of the patient."

As we touched on earlier, this is important from a clinical and marketing sense. Within the appropriate HIPPA laws you should update the primary care physician or referring physician upon evaluation and discharge/referral. This not only offers the patient a complete health record, but also gets your name in front of the physician in a professional and courteous fashion. The case notes can simply include the initial date of service, patient name, diagnosis, and current treatment plan, unless additional information is requested.

Hinderance to Chiropractic Referral #3-
Chiropractors "Steal" patients while attempting to
treat outside of their scope

Your Position Statement- "We are not a primary care office and we believe that co-management and interdisciplinary communication are essential to optimal patient outcomes."

Some physicians are leery that "chiropractors try to treat everything" and may be concerned about your "stealing" their patients. Just simply let the physician know that you work with quite a few primary care offices in town and your focus is on neuro-musculoskeletal care. We know that chiropractic care may have an impact on health conditions beyond simply neuro-musculoskeltal complaints. However, with this conversation you need to stay focused on your message and your marketing. You may have only a few minutes with the doctor and attempting to explain every condition which chiropractic care can help is an impossible task. As your relationship develops you will be able to touch an a variety of conditions.

These are the 3 big hurdles that many MD's have when first referring a patient to a chiropractor. It is best to address them up front. You want to make sure the physician aware that you do everything possible to make referrals easy and quick. Depending upon your volume and office structure you can promote that referred patients are seen same day, within 24 hours, or within 48 hours. Also, be sure to let them know that chiropractic coverage is available on most insurance plans as illustrated on your Practice Information Sheet.

You have covered most of the imperative topics at this point. If the physician has additional interest in safety and efficacy with certain conditions you can discuss these topics and pull the research from your previously prepared folder.

The bottom line is that our biggest perceived "competition" for these referrals is physical therapy and NSAID's. In reality, we really have no competition because our service is unique, effective, and safe. It is most important to expose these medical doctor's to the unique aspects of chiropractic and helping them understand the service which we offer. Statistically, the traditional protocols of spine care are woefully inadequate, but, as we know, it's very difficult to change a habit! This is no different for referrals; and this is why consistent, positive, educational and motivational outreach is the key to building this relationship.

Finishing up, it's always important to let that doctor know that, as a trusted referral partner, he can expect to receive a monthly research brief from you highlighting an important study in musculoskeletal care.

Some chiropractors become concerned that their monthly outreach through research may end up in the circular file. I have found a great way to insure that your future correspondence reaches the doctor is to directly address this with the front desk staff on your way out of the office. Thank the front desk staff and let him/her know that their physician will be expecting monthly research updates from your office. Let them know to keep any eye out for an envelope with your practice information around the first of each month. This emphasizes the importance of the upcoming correspondence and they will be sure the doctor gets the research updates if they know he/ she will be expecting it!

CHAPTER NINE
Delivering Value Over Time

Immediately upon leaving the office, its good practice to promptly open your tracking sheet and input the names of employees, your general feelings regarding the meeting, and any other notes you may have while they are fresh.

This would include if the doctor asked for research which you did not have readily present. I recommend following up with this research within a week. Also, if the doctor asked some specific questions regarding technique or condition specific treatment, then I would be sure to mark this down on your tracking sheet. This way you will be able to find some research and surprise him/her with a it shortly after your visit.

Your gut feeling on the meeting is also important. Marking this down will help you as time progresses on. If you had a great meeting but do not see any referred patients, then you may have just missed a key point. For doctors whom you established great rapport, it will be easy to them give them a call and follow up.

It's important to do this directly after you leave the office because most of the information will be forgotten in the next 30-45 minutes unless you write it down. This tracking sheet provides your blueprint for further communication. When you follow up and are able to address the staff by name it will make a huge impact. You should always strive to provide a personal touch with your outreach. It does not go unnoticed and it will further position yourself within your community.

Following up consistently is perhaps the biggest pitfall of chiropractors that I work with. With the hard work of producing your MD list, verifying your MD list, and finishing up your MD meeting, the follow through is the easy part. It should take minimal time, effort, and cost. However, the time and money that is used will be well spent.

I recommend following up with our MD Follow Up Letter within the next week. This letter reinforces your visit and continues to set the stage for further communication. While there is no "magic" in the individual steps listed in this book, it is truly the complete package of outreach which will create the most impact. Then you will need to simply follow up with evaluation/discharge notes for each patient and your monthly MD Research Briefs.

Remember, habits (referral or personal) are hard to break. It will take consistent communication for you to establish yourself as their first choice for musculoskeletal care. Once you begin to receive referrals from a variety of MD's in your area it will greatly impact your practice and provide you with exposure that many chiropractors do not yet have.

As time progresses you may notice that some physicians on your list have not referred a patient to your office. I recommend a few months of outreach before following up and contacting the physician, but there are no firm guides for the amount of time you should let elapse before following up. It is best to follow up directly over the phone. Below is a sample script.

"Hello Dr. Smith, this is Dr. Langmaid at ABC Spine Clinic. You should be receiving our monthly research updates on musculoskeletal care which we discussed during our meeting. I noticed that we have seen limited referrals from your practice. During our meeting you mentioned that you see a significant amount patients presenting with spine complaints daily in practice. Are there any specific conditions or areas of interest where I can provide additional information?"

At this point, simply listen. The doctor will either provide you with an answer on some specific conditions of interest or he will let you know why he is not currently referring to your office. This information is extremely valuable because it will help you refine your MD Target List. If you get the feeling that the doctor is avoiding the question or provides a limited response, then you may entertain the idea of removing him from you list. However, it may just be a simple phone call reminder which stimulates the relationship. Either way, the act of following up with contribute to the efficiency of your physician outreach.

To improve the efficiency of your outreach it is important to create multiple "touches" per month to the physicians practice. This includes your MD Case Notes, you monthly MD Research Brief, and then periodic personal outreach. If you are able to reach out through a variety of different means, it will improve the likelihood that the physician will not only come to recognize and remember your name, but he/she will also begin to identify that you are the local expert on musculoskeletal care. As you establish yourself as the expert, you will become the obvious choice for referrals.

Everything in this guide should be used a guideline for your communication. It was developed from research articles (regarding who, what, and where MD's are referring) and my personal experience building a referral based practice. Feel free to customize the content for your personal practice. Every chiropractor practices slightly different and you should use the opportunity to meet with MD's as a vehicle to promote, establish, and enhance relationships through an authentic and elegant program which begins with you!

CHAPTER TEN
Engage, Educate, and Entertain

Keep in mind your MD List should be a dynamic set of physicians in your area. Roughly 1-5% of your list will turn over each quarter. This may be due to the physician moving or jointing another practice. Also, as you follow through with your MD Meetings, you will gain knowledge and an understanding of each physicians practice. Transitioning non-referring doctors off of your list will be something that you should explore every few months.

Another great low cost way to interact and meet up with local physicians is at Grand Rounds at your local hospital. Nearly every hospital hosts spine specific Grand Rounds either weekly or monthly. These meetings offer an opportunity to learn about their practices', build rapport, and perhaps even obtain continuing education credits (depending upon the state). To find out if your local hospital hosts grand rounds simply call and ask. If they do not, typically they can direct you to a local hospital that does.

In my experience Grand Rounds usually consist of various surgeons, physicians assistants, hospital administrators, radiologists, and surgical implant representatives. The surgical implant companies typically sponsor the event and food is usually provided. Often, the meetings will consist of a presentation on a specific topic which is following by case conferences on individual cases/films which the attendees bring. Not only is the knowledge you can obtain at these events worth its weight in gold, but you are also able to interact and expose other health professionals to your practice. Additionally, you will get a myriad of "inside information" regarding spine procedures, orthopedic technique, hospital policies/procedures, etc. which you can then share with your patients. I cannot overstate the value and exposure you can get from these meetings. Learning about the current trends and advancements in the treatment of spine related complaints will give you a huge edge when communicating with your patients and other providers. I have been fortunate to actually present at a hospital for continuing education credits for medical doctors. To date, very few chiropractors have presented for CEU's to medial doctors. This trend will hopefully change as more chiropractors become involved at their local spine conference and grand round programs.

Using social media to expose your local community and patients to advances in research is also a great idea. It is low cost and can be highly effective. An important consideration when using social media is your POSITIONING. Many physicians have greatly compromised their integrity and reputation due to poor choices across various social media platforms. I strongly encourage you to keep your communication professional at all times. One of the easiest ways to do this is to focus on research. By focusing on research you are able to position yourself appropriately while also avoiding any topics which may come off in poor taste. A simple, straightforward, professionally designed page with consistent content is a step in the right direction.

Pages such as The Evidence Based Chiropractor offer free daily content which can be shared on your practice page. Social media outlets such as Facebook allow a variety of advertising options for your page. These should be carefully considered before any investment is made. Targeting, CTR, copyrighting, testing, photo choice, and a variety of other factors can make a campaign either extremely successful or an absolute failure. Carefully analyzing your return on investment and setting up a campaign to increase your mailing list through the promotion of landing pages can yield great results if done properly. If you do choose to participate in some paid advertising, I recommend enlisting professional help. Obtaining help will assist you in refining your goals and creating a campaign that will maximize your budget. There are a variety of social media experts (in and out of chiropractic) available. It is best to determine your goals with social media first. It may be to increase your fan base, spread a message of conservative health care, build your mailing list, or even directly solicit new patients. Your goals will determine who or what social media organization can best address your needs. This enables you to interview and work with a team that can focus and create the best ROI for your project.

CHAPTER ELEVEN
In Closing

Building a referral-based practice is the easiest way to insure you are able to not only stay afloat, but prosper, during the turbulent seas of increased deductibles, exorbitant co-pays, and government intervention into healthcare. By establishing yourself as the premier conservative option for musculoskeletal care in your area; you will be able to retain a steady stream of new patients from other physicians. It is important to keep in mind that research and evidence based practice guidelines support referrals for chiropractic care. Reaching out to other physicians should not be viewed as "soliciting" patients; but rather availing yourself as the local expert in the care which their patients need.

The transition of our payment model from care based upon the number of interventions towards care based upon outcomes is already under way. The new ICD-10 coding will greatly enhance the third party payers' ability to establish specific data and "trends" of care, which will inevitably drive reimbursement. The wealth of research supporting the efficacy and safety of chiropractic care will also be of greater importance as we move through this health care transition. We, as a profession, must promote and push this research to the forefront and those of us which already have these referral relationships in place will have a distinct advantage in our local markets.

While the thought of starting an interdisciplinary outreach process can seem intimidating at first, you will find that it is very straightforward using a systematic approach. Presenting and positioning yourself in an elegant and professional manner will reap rewards and help establish relationships for years to come. Not relying on the expensive and every changing legality of public advertising will benefit your practice in many ways. The relationships you establish with local physicians should last years and result in potentially hundreds of patients referred to your office.

The last generation of chiropractors laid the groundwork for the swell of chiropractic research which is being produced. The importance of this contribution cannot be overstated. Even though our market penetration did not climb during this time, they provided a framework from which our "niche" profession can reach a mass audience and perhaps push over the tipping point. Our generation must take the reigns and build the interdisciplinary relationships which will insure the unique nature of our practice is able to further penetrate into the healthcare marketplace.

Positioning yourself as an evidence based chiropractor that has deep relationships with other health professionals is a great way to ensure practice success in the coming years. Fortunately, research continues to show that chiropractic care is one of the best options for conservative care for a vast variety of conditions. From randomized controlled trials, to best practices and evidence-based care guidelines, chiropractic research is making an impact across the board. However, the onus is on us to promote this research and build the relationships necessary to create referrals. These referrals are not merely for the benefit of your practice, but also truly for the benefits of these patients. Chiropractic care continues to be considered a safe and effective health profession. The art, science, and philosophy of chiropractic will continue to evolve and refine itself. Holistic and conservative care have unprecedented support and interest from the public and other health professionals. It has never been a better time to be a chiropractor!.

ABOUT THE AUTHOR

Dr. Jeff Langmaid is an internationally recognized author, speaker, and chiropractor. He is the founder of The Evidence Based Chiropractor LLC, an organization dedicated to increasing chiropractic utilization. A thought-leader regarding interdisciplinary communication, practice, and marketing; he has been heralded as one of chiropractic's new innovators. He has been featured on Yahoo Health, Prevention, and by CBS News. You can find him where chiropractic care, creative design, and Healthcare 2.0 meet.

TheEvidenceBasedChiropractor.com

ACKNOWLEDGMENTS

Sara Langmaid, John Apsey, Caitlyn Fick, Marti Martin, Walter and Barbara Langmaid, Paul Friemel, TJ Mapes, Michael Poorman, Neville Medhora, all members and friends of The Evidence Based Chiropractor

Thank you- Seth Godin, Guy Riekeman, Reggie Gold, Marc Ecko, Simon Sinek, and Paul Arden for the inspiration.

The Evidence Based Chiropractor is the worldwide leader in chiropractic communication and marketing. Our service is dedicated to increasing chiropractic utilization by showcasing research. Marketing through research is efficient, cost effective, and can dramatically improve your incoming referrals. Join us. Lets grow chiropractic together.

Visit our Store to see our full line of chiropractic products and services.

Made in the USA
San Bernardino, CA
14 February 2016